A

▼ IV FACTS

Preparation: Do not use PVC container if infusion is to exceed 2 hr; use glass or polyolefin instead. Dilute 150 mg in 100 mL D₅W for rapid loading dose (1.5 mg/mL). Dilute 900 mg in 500 mL D₅W for slow infusions (1.8 mg/mL). Store at room temperature and use within 24 hr.

Infusion: Infuse loading dose over 10 min. Immediately follow with slow infusion of 1 mg/min or 33.3 mL/hr. Maintenance infusion of 0.5 mg/min or 16.6 mL/hr can be continued up to 96 hr. Use of an infusion pump is advised.

Incompatibilities: Do not mix with aminophylline, cefazolin, heparin, sodium bicarbonate; do not mix in solution with other drugs.

Adverse effects

- **CNS:** *Malaise, fatigue, dizziness, tremors, ataxia,* paresthesias, lack of coordination
- **CV: Cardiac arrhythmias,** heart failure, **cardiac arrest,** hypotension, bradycardia
- **EENT:** *Corneal microdeposits* (photophobia, dry eyes, halos, blurred vision); ophthalmic abnormalities including permanent blindness
- **Endocrine:** *Hypothyroidism or hyperthyroidism*
- **GI:** *Nausea, vomiting, anorexia, constipation, abnormal LFT,* **hepatotox**...
- **Respiratory: Pulmonary toxicit**... pneumonitis, infiltrates (shortnes... breath, cough, rales, wheezes)
- **Other:** *Photosensitivity,* angioedema, fe...

Interactions

❋ **Drug- drug** • Increased digitalis toxici... with digoxin • Increased risk of rhabdomyolysis if combined with simvastatin; limit simvastatin to less than 20 mg/dose • Increased quinidine toxicity with quinidine • Increased flecainide toxicity with amiodarone • Increased risk of arrhythmias with azole antifungals, fluoroquinolones, macrolide antibiotics, ranolazine, trazodone, thioridazine, vardenafil, ziprasidone • Increased phenytoin toxicity with phenytoin, ethotoin • Increased bleeding tendencies with warfarin • Potential sinus arrest and heart block with beta-blockers, calcium channel blockers

❋ **Drug-lab test** • Increased T₄ levels, increased serum reverse T₃ levels

❋ **Drug-food** • Increased risk of toxicit... oral form combined with grapefruit juice; avoid this combination

■ Nursing considerations

CLINICAL ALERT!
Name confusion has occurred with amrinone (name has now been changed to inamrinone, but confusion may still occur); use caution.

Assessment

- **History:** Hypersensitivity to amiodaron... sinus node dysfunction, heart block, seve... bradycardia, hypokalemia, lactation, th... roid dysfunction, pregnancy
- **Physical:** Skin color, lesions; reflexes, ga... eye examination; P, BP, auscultation, co... tinuous ECG monitoring; R, adventitio... sounds, baseline chest X-ray; liver evalu... tion; LFTs, serum electrolytes, T₄, and T3...

Interventions

⊗ ***Black box warning*** Reserve use fo... life-threatening arrhythmias; serious toxic... ty, including arrhythmias, pulmonary toxic... ity can occur.
- Monitor cardiac rhythm...
- Monit...

...grapefruit juice while on this drug.
- Have regular medical follow-up, moni-...

2014
LIPPINCOTT'S
Nursing
Drug Guide

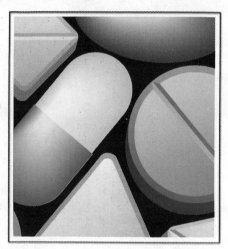

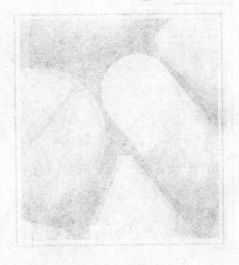

2014
LIPPINCOTT'S
Nursing
Drug Guide

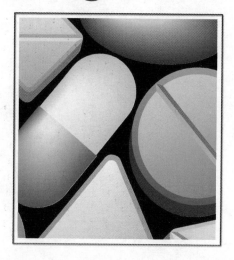

A

▼ IV FACTS

Preparation: Do not use PVC container if infusion is to exceed 2 hr; use glass or polyolefin instead. Dilute 150 mg in 100 mL D₅W for rapid loading dose (1.5 mg/mL). Dilute 900 mg in 500 mL D₅W for slow infusions (1.8 mg/mL). Store at room temperature and use within 24 hr.

Infusion: Infuse loading dose over 10 min. Immediately follow with slow infusion of 1 mg/min or 33.3 mL/hr. Maintenance infusion of 0.5 mg/min or 16.6 mL/hr can be continued up to 96 hr. Use of an infusion pump is advised.

Incompatibilities: Do not mix with aminophylline, cefazolin, heparin, sodium bicarbonate; do not mix in solution with other drugs.

✱ Drug-food • Increased risk of toxicity if oral form combined with grapefruit juice; avoid this combination

■ Nursing considerations

CLINICAL ALERT!
Name confusion has occurred with amrinone (name has now been changed to inamrinone, but confusion may still occur); use caution.

Assessment
- **History:** Hypersensitivity to amiodarone, sinus node dysfunction, heart block, severe bradycardia, hypokalemia, lactation, thyroid dysfunction, pregnancy
- **Physical:** Skin color, lesions; reflexes, gait, eye examination; P, BP, auscultation, continuous ECG monitoring; R, adventitious sounds, baseline chest X-ray; liver evaluation; LFTs, serum electrolytes, T₄, and T₃

Interventions
⊗ **Black box warning** Reserve use for life-threatening arrhythmias; serious toxicity, including arrhythmias, pulmonary toxicity can occur.
- Monitor cardiac rhythm continuously.
- Monitor for an extended period when dosage adjustments are made.
⊗ **Warning** Monitor for safe and effective serum levels (0.5–2.5 mcg/mL).
⊗ **Warning** Doses of digoxin, quinidine, phenytoin, and warfarin may need to be reduced one-third to one-half when amiodarone is started.

Teaching points
- Drug dosage will be changed in relation to response of arrhythmias; you will need to be hospitalized during initiation of drug therapy; you will be closely monitored when dosage is changed.
- Avoid grapefruit juice while on this drug.
- Have regular medical follow-up, moni-

Adverse effects
- **CNS:** *Malaise, fatigue, dizziness, tremors, ataxia,* paresthesias, lack of coordination
- **CV:** **Cardiac arrhythmias,** heart failure, **cardiac arrest,** hypotension, bradycardia
- **EENT:** *Corneal microdeposits* (photophobia, dry eyes, halos, blurred vision); ophthalmic abnormalities including permanent blindness
- **Endocrine:** *Hypothyroidism or hyperthyroidism*
- **GI:** *Nausea, vomiting, anorexia, constipation, abnormal LFT,* **hepatotoxicity**
- **Respiratory:** **Pulmonary toxicity**—pneumonitis, infiltrates (shortness of breath, cough, rales, wheezes)
- **Other:** *Photosensitivity,* angioedema, fever

Interactions
✱ Drug-drug • Increased digitalis toxicity with digoxin • Increased risk of rhabdomyolysis if combined with simvastatin; limit simvastatin to less than 20 mg/dose • Increased quinidine toxicity with quinidine • Increased flecainide toxicity with amiodarone • Increased risk of arrhythmias with azole antifungals, fluoroquinolones, macrolide antibiotics, ranolazine, trazodone, thioridazine, vardenafil, ziprasidone • Increased phenytoin toxicity with phenytoin, ethotoin • Increased bleeding tendencies with warfarin • Potential sinus arrest and heart block with beta-blockers, calcium channel blockers
✱ Drug-lab test • Increased T₄ levels, increased serum reverse T₃ levels

D1005280